BLEEDING PILES REMEDIES

"DIAGNOSIS, EXPLORING PREVENTION, AND HOLISTIC APPROACHES TO STOP HEMORRHOID BLEEDING"

BY

BOFEST JOYFUL

COPYRIGHT

COPYRIGHT © 2023 BY JOYFUL BOFEST

TABLE OF CONTENTS

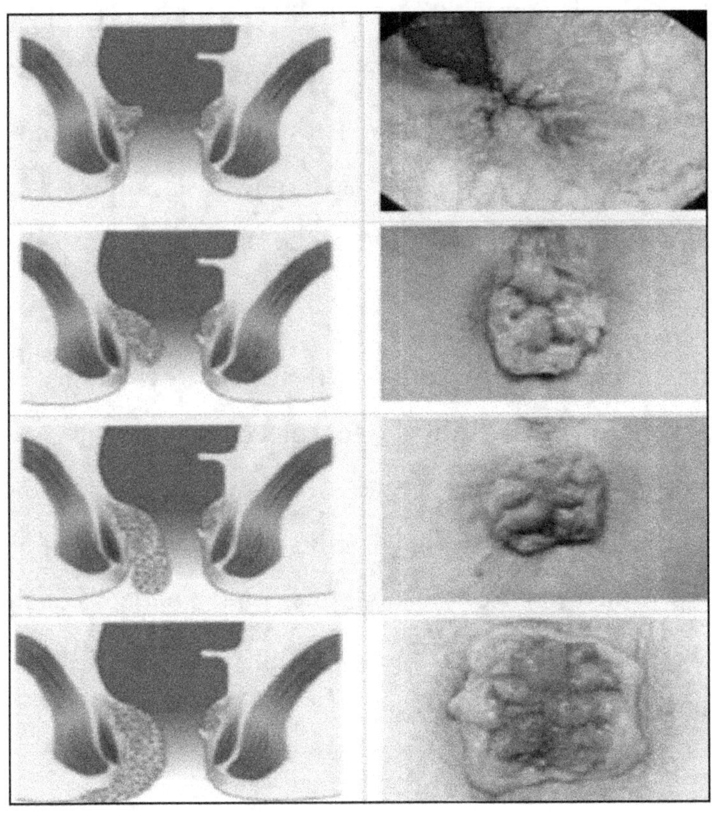

INTRODUCTION

Bleeding Piles Unveiled: Exploring Hemorrhoidal Hemorrhage

Welcome to "Bleeding Piles Unveiled: Exploring Hemorrhoidal Hemorrhage", an in-depth analysis of one of the most common yet misunderstood medical conditions in the world. Hemorrhoids, also known as piles, affect millions of people across the globe and can cause severe discomfort and embarrassment.

In this book, we will delve into the causes, symptoms, and treatment options available for bleeding piles. We will explore the various types of hemorrhoids, their classification, and how they can be prevented. We will also examine the effects of bleeding piles on the patient's quality of life and provide solutions on how to mitigate and manage the condition.

Whether you are a healthcare provider, a patient suffering from hemorrhoidal hemorrhage, or simply interested in learning more about this condition, "Bleeding Piles Unveiled: Exploring Hemorrhoidal Hemorrhage" is the ultimate guide for you. With expert insights, practical tips, and real-life case studies, this book will equip you with the knowledge and tools you need to effectively tackle bleeding piles and improve your overall well-being.

CHAPTER ONE

THE ANATOMY OF HEMORRHOIDS: UNDERSTANDING THE NATURE OF BLEEDING PILES

Hemorrhoids are vascular structures in the anal canal that help with Hemorrhoids are vascular structures in the anal canal that help with stool control. When they become swollen or inflamed, they can cause discomfort, pain, and bleeding. Here's an overview of their anatomy:

TYPES OF HEMORRHOIDS:
Internal Hemorrhoids:

Located inside the rectum, usually painless unless they prolapse (extend outside the anus).

Covered by a mucous membrane, which lacks pain receptors, so bleeding might be the primary symptom.

External Hemorrhoids:

Form under the skin around the anus.

Often more painful as they have numerous pain receptors.

ANATOMY OF HEMORRHOIDS:

Blood Vessels:

Hemorrhoids consist of blood vessels, supporting tissue, and muscle fibers.

They have a network of small arteries and veins that can become engorged and swollen, leading to the development of hemorrhoids.

Supporting Tissue:

Made up of connective tissue and elastin fibers that help maintain the structure of the hemorrhoidal cushions.

Location:

- Found at the junction where the rectum and anus meet.

- Internal hemorrhoids originate above the dentate line (where the sensitive skin transitions to the less sensitive lining of the rectum).

- External hemorrhoids develop below the dentate line and have more pain receptors.

Muscle Fibers:

Smooth muscle fibers in the walls of blood vessels and surrounding tissues help regulate blood flow and contraction.

CAUSES OF HEMORRHOIDS:
Strain During Bowel Movements:

Constipation or excessive straining during bowel movements can increase pressure on the rectal veins, leading to hemorrhoids.

Pregnancy:

Increased pressure on the pelvic veins due to the growing uterus can cause hemorrhoids in pregnant women.

Chronic Diarrhea or Constipation:

Both can contribute to the development of hemorrhoids by putting strain on the rectal area.

Obesity:

Being overweight can increase the likelihood of developing hemorrhoids due to increased pressure on the rectal veins.

TREATMENT:
Lifestyle Changes:

Consuming a high-fiber diet, staying hydrated, and avoiding prolonged sitting or straining during bowel movements can alleviate symptoms.

Medications:

Over-the-counter creams, ointments, or suppositories can relieve pain and itching.

Medical Procedures:
If conservative measures fail, procedures like rubber band ligation, sclerotherapy, infrared coagulation, or surgical removal may be necessary.

Bleeding piles, also known as bleeding hemorrhoids, occur when the swollen or inflamed blood vessels in the anal canal rupture or tear, resulting in bleeding. Understanding the nature of bleeding piles involves several aspects:

CAUSES OF BLEEDING PILES:

Strain during Bowel Movements:

Excessive straining during bowel movements can put pressure on the hemorrhoidal veins, leading to bleeding.

Hard Stools/Constipation:

Passing hard stools can irritate hemorrhoids and cause bleeding.

Chronic Diarrhea:

Frequent and prolonged episodes of diarrhea can also contribute to the development or worsening of bleeding piles.

Pregnancy:

Increased pressure on the pelvic area during pregnancy can cause hemorrhoids, leading to bleeding.

NATURE OF BLEEDING:
Color of Blood:

Bleeding from hemorrhoids typically presents as bright red blood on the stool, toilet paper, or in the toilet bowl.

Amount of Bleeding:

The amount of bleeding can vary, from small streaks to more significant amounts. Heavy bleeding might indicate other conditions and requires medical attention.

Associated Symptoms:

Bleeding piles might be accompanied by itching, pain, discomfort, or a feeling of fullness in the anal area.

DIAGNOSIS AND TREATMENT:
Physical Examination:

A doctor can diagnose bleeding piles by conducting a physical examination of the anal area.

Stool Test or Colonoscopy:

In some cases, a stool test or colonoscopy may be recommended to rule out other causes of bleeding, especially if there's a concern about other gastrointestinal issues.

Treatment:

Treatment often involves lifestyle modifications like a high-fiber diet, increased fluid intake, and avoiding straining during bowel movements.

Over-the-counter creams, ointments, or suppositories can help reduce symptoms.

Medical procedures like rubber band ligation, sclerotherapy, or surgical removal might be necessary for severe cases.

When to Seek Medical Help:
Excessive Bleeding:

If bleeding is heavy or persistent, medical attention is crucial to rule out more serious conditions.

Severe Pain or Discomfort:

Persistent pain or discomfort despite home remedies should prompt a visit to a healthcare professional.

Understanding the anatomy of hemorrhoids helps in managing symptoms and seeking appropriate treatment. However, if you're experiencing severe pain, bleeding, or persistent symptoms, consulting a healthcare professional is crucial for proper diagnosis and treatment.

CHAPTER TWO

SYMPTOMS DECODED: RECOGNIZING AND ADDRESSING HEMORRHOID BLEEDING

Hemorrhoids are swollen veins in the lowest part of your rectum and anus, and bleeding is a common symptom. Here's some guidance on how to recognize and address it:

RECOGNIZING HEMORRHOID BLEEDING:

Blood in Stool: You might notice blood on your toilet paper, in the toilet bowl, or on the stool itself after a bowel movement.

Bright Red Blood: Bleeding from hemorrhoids often appears bright red since it comes from veins close to the anus.

Addressing Hemorrhoid Bleeding:

Consult a Doctor: If you notice bleeding, especially if it's recurrent, consult a healthcare professional. They can diagnose the issue and suggest appropriate treatment.

HOME REMEDIES:

Dietary Changes: Increase fiber intake to soften stools and ease bowel movements.

Hydration: Drink plenty of water to prevent constipation.

Topical Treatments: Over-the-counter creams or ointments may help relieve symptoms.

Warm Baths: Soaking in warm water can soothe the area.

MEDICAL TREATMENTS:

Medications: Your doctor may prescribe medications to reduce swelling or recommend suppositories to ease discomfort.

Procedures: In severe cases, procedures like rubber band ligation, sclerotherapy, or surgery might be necessary.

PREVENTIVE MEASURES:

Maintain Good Bowel Habits: Avoid straining during bowel movements and try not to sit on the toilet for too long.

Healthy Lifestyle: Exercise regularly and maintain a healthy weight to prevent excessive pressure on the veins in the lower rectum.

Avoid Aggravating Factors: Limit prolonged sitting, especially on hard surfaces, and be mindful of heavy lifting.

CHAPTER THREE

DIAGNOSTIC TECHNIQUES AND TOOLS: UNVEILING THE BLEEDING PILES' TRUTH

Physical Examination: During a physical exam, the doctor inspects the anal area for external hemorrhoids, swelling, or signs of irritation. They might also look for internal hemorrhoids that protrude outside the anus during straining.

Anoscopy: This involves inserting a small, tubular instrument (anoscope) into the anus to visualize internal hemorrhoids. It allows direct inspection of the anal canal and lower rectum, revealing the presence, size, and location of hemorrhoids.

Proctoscopy: Similar to anoscope, proctoscopy employs a longer, flexible instrument (proctoscope) to examine the rectum. It offers a more comprehensive view of the rectal lining, allowing for a detailed assessment of hemorrhoids and other abnormalities.

Colonoscopy: While primarily used to examine the entire colon for various conditions, colonoscopy can detect internal hemorrhoids located higher up in the rectum. It helps rule out other potential causes of rectal bleeding.

Sigmoidoscopy: Focusing on the lower part of the colon and rectum, sigmoidoscopy aids in identifying bleeding sources such as internal hemorrhoids and inflammation.

Digital Rectal Examination (DRE): By inserting a lubricated, gloved finger into the rectum, the doctor can feel for abnormalities like swollen blood vessels (hemorrhoids), fissures, or other rectal issues.

Stool Examination: This involves analyzing stool samples for the presence of blood, which could indicate bleeding from hemorrhoids or other gastrointestinal conditions.

Blood Tests: Blood tests check for anemia or infections, common in individuals experiencing prolonged bleeding from hemorrhoids.

Ultrasound: Using sound waves, ultrasound can produce images to identify the presence and size of hemorrhoids, especially those located internally.

MRI (Magnetic Resonance Imaging): MRI provides detailed images of the pelvic area, aiding in the identification and assessment of hemorrhoids and associated complications.

CT Scan (Computed Tomography): CT scans offer cross-sectional images for a comprehensive evaluation of the rectal area, helping detect hemorrhoids and ruling out other conditions.

Transrectal Ultrasound (TRUS): This imaging technique specifically examines the rectum and surrounding structures using sound waves, providing detailed images to detect and assess hemorrhoids.

Colonography (Virtual Colonoscopy): Offering a detailed picture of the colon and rectum, this technique aids in detecting and evaluating hemorrhoids and other colorectal issues.

Endorectal Ultrasound (ERUS): ERUS provides detailed imaging of the rectal area, helping identify hemorrhoids and assess their severity.

Flexible Sigmoidoscopy: Similar to colonoscopy, this technique focuses on the rectum and lower colon, aiding in the identification and assessment of bleeding sources.

Rectal Manometry: This technique measures the pressure and reflexes of the anal sphincter muscles and rectum, assisting in diagnosing conditions like hemorrhoids.

Angiography: Using X-rays to visualize blood vessels, angiography helps identify the source of bleeding in hemorrhoids or other vascular conditions.

Biopsy: Taking tissue samples for microscopic examination helps rule out other conditions that may mimic hemorrhoids, ensuring an accurate diagnosis.

Capsule Endoscopy: By capturing images as it travels through the digestive tract, this method can identify bleeding sources in the colon and rectum, including hemorrhoids.

Colon Transit Study: Evaluating the movement of stool through the colon helps identify abnormalities contributing to bleeding, including hemorrhoids.

CHAPTER FOUR

PREVENTION PROTOCOLS: STRATEGIES TO AVOID HEMORRHOID BLEEDING

Preventing hemorrhoid bleeding involves several strategies aimed at reducing strain on the rectal area and minimizing irritation. Here are some effective prevention protocols:

Dietary Modifications:

High-Fiber Diet: Include foods such as whole grains (brown rice, oatmeal), fruits (apples, berries), vegetables (broccoli, spinach), and legumes (beans, lentils) in your meals. Fiber supplements like psyllium husk can also be beneficial.

Adequate Hydration: Aim for at least 8 cups (64 ounces) of water daily. Hydration keeps stools soft and facilitates their movement through the digestive tract.

Healthy Bowel Habits:

Regular Bowel Movements: Establish a routine by trying to use the restroom around the same time each day. Having meals rich in fiber can help stimulate regular bowel movements.

Avoid Straining: If you feel the need to strain during bowel movements, it might indicate constipation. Consider stool softeners or gentle laxatives after consulting a healthcare professional.

Good Toilet Habits:

Avoid Prolonged Sitting: Try not to sit on the toilet for extended periods. If you find yourself unable to pass stool, it's better to leave and try again later.

Use Soft Toilet Paper: Opt for unscented, dye-free, and soft toilet paper to prevent further irritation. Consider using wet wipes for a more thorough and gentle cleaning.

Lifestyle Changes:

Regular Exercise: Engage in activities like walking, swimming, or yoga to improve blood circulation and promote regular bowel movements.

Weight Management: Excess weight, especially around the abdomen, can increase pressure on the rectal area. Maintaining a healthy weight reduces strain on hemorrhoids.

Proper Hygiene:

Gentle Cleaning: Use lukewarm water or unscented, alcohol-free wipes to cleanse the area after bowel movements. Pat the area dry with a soft towel instead of rubbing.

Avoid Harsh Cleansers: Refrain from using soaps or cleansers with fragrances or harsh chemicals, as they can irritate the sensitive skin around hemorrhoids.

Medical Interventions:

Topical Treatments: Over-the-counter creams containing hydrocortisone or witch hazel can help alleviate itching and discomfort. Apply as directed by the product label or a healthcare professional.

Consultation with a Doctor: If bleeding persists or worsens, seek medical advice promptly. Your doctor might recommend prescription medications, procedures like rubber band ligation, sclerotherapy, or surgery in severe cases.

Avoidance of Aggravating Factors:

Limit Straining Activities: Avoid activities that involve heavy lifting or straining, as they can exacerbate hemorrhoid symptoms. If lifting is necessary, use proper techniques and avoid holding your breath.

Manage Chronic Conditions: Conditions like irritable bowel syndrome (IBS), Crohn's disease, or ulcerative colitis can affect bowel movements and worsen hemorrhoids. Follow treatment plans recommended by your healthcare provider to manage these conditions effectively.

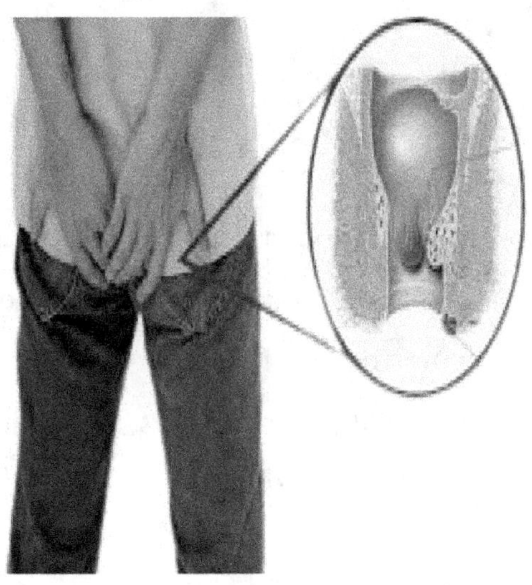

CHAPTER FIVE

MEDICAL INTERVENTIONS: MODERN TREATMENTS FOR HEMORRHOIDAL HEMORRHAGE

Hemorrhoidal bleeding, often associated with hemorrhoids, can be distressing and uncomfortable. There are various modern medical interventions available to address hemorrhoidal hemorrhage, ranging from conservative measures to more invasive treatments, depending on the severity and nature of the condition.

Home Remedies and Conservative Treatments:
Dietary Modifications: Increasing fiber intake through fruits, vegetables, and whole grains can soften stools and

reduce straining during bowel movements, easing hemorrhoidal bleeding.

Topical Treatments: Over-the-counter creams, ointments, and suppositories containing hydrocortisone or witch hazel can help alleviate symptoms like itching and pain.

Sitz Baths: Soaking the affected area in warm water for 10-15 minutes several times a day can provide relief and promote healing.

Minimally Invasive Procedures:
Rubber Band Ligation: This procedure involves placing a rubber band around the base of the hemorrhoid to cut off its blood supply. Eventually, the hemorrhoid shrinks and falls off.

Sclerotherapy: A solution is injected into the hemorrhoid, causing it to shrink and eventually disappear.

Infrared Coagulation: A probe is used to expose the hemorrhoidal tissue to infrared light, which coagulates the blood vessels, causing the hemorrhoid to shrink.

Surgical Interventions:

Hemorrhoidectomy: In severe cases or when other treatments have failed, a surgical procedure to remove the hemorrhoids may be recommended. Traditional hemorrhoidectomy involves excising the hemorrhoids using a scalpel, while newer techniques like stapled hemorrhoidopexy or Doppler-guided hemorrhoidal artery ligation (HAL) aim to reduce pain and recovery time.

Laser Treatment: Ablation or vaporization of hemorrhoidal tissue using a laser can be employed to remove or shrink hemorrhoids.

Emerging Treatments:

Transanal Hemorrhoidal Dearterialization (THD): This minimally invasive procedure uses an ultrasound to locate the arteries supplying blood to the hemorrhoids, which are then ligated to reduce blood flow and shrink the hemorrhoids.

Radiofrequency Ablation (RFA): Applying radiofrequency energy to the hemorrhoidal tissue can cause coagulation and subsequent shrinkage of the hemorrhoids.

Cryotherapy: Freezing the hemorrhoidal tissue can cause it to shrink and alleviate symptoms.

Lifestyle Modifications:

Hydration and Exercise: Drinking an adequate amount of water and engaging in regular physical activity can promote regular bowel movements, reducing the strain on hemorrhoids.

Avoiding Prolonged Sitting or Straining: Sitting for extended periods and straining during bowel movements can exacerbate hemorrhoidal bleeding. Taking breaks and avoiding excessive straining is crucial.

CHAPTER SIX

HOLISTIC HEALING APPROACHES: NATURAL REMEDIES AND LIFESTYLE CHANGES

Holistic healing emphasizes treating the whole person—mind, body, and spirit—rather than just addressing specific symptoms or ailments. Natural remedies and lifestyle changes play a significant role in holistic healing approaches. Here are some common practices:Natural Remedies:

Herbal Medicine:

Herbs and Plants: These have been used for centuries across cultures for their medicinal properties. For instance, ginseng is known for energy enhancement, while chamomile helps with relaxation and sleep.

Essential Oils: Derived from plants, these oils offer various benefits. Lavender is popular for calming effects, peppermint for headaches, and tea tree for its antimicrobial properties.

Nutritional Therapy:

Dietary Changes: Whole foods provide essential nutrients, antioxidants, and fiber vital for optimal health. Emphasizing a rainbow of fruits and vegetables ensures a diverse range of nutrients.

Supplements: They're used to address specific deficiencies or health concerns. Vitamin D for bone health or omega-3 fatty acids for heart health are common examples.

Traditional Medicine:

TCM: Acupuncture stimulates specific points on the body to promote energy flow and alleviate ailments. Tai chi and qi gong, on the other hand, focus on movement, breath, and energy cultivation for overall health.

Ayurveda: This system emphasizes finding balance among different body types or doshas. It utilizes specific diets, herbal treatments, and practices like yoga to achieve harmony.

Lifestyle Changes:

Mindfulness and Stress Reduction:

Meditation: Beyond stress reduction, it improves focus, emotional well-being, and even physical health by reducing inflammation and enhancing immune function.

Yoga: Combining physical postures (asanas), breath control (pranayama), and meditation, it fosters flexibility, strength, and mental calmness.

Physical Activity:

Exercise: Regular physical activity not only boosts cardiovascular health but also aids in maintaining healthy weight, improving mood, and reducing the risk of chronic diseases.

Holistic Therapies:

Massage Therapy: It's not just about relaxation; it can ease muscle tension, improve circulation, and reduce stress hormones like cortisol.

Chiropractic Care: By aligning the spine and musculoskeletal system, it aims to improve nervous system function and overall health.

Energy Healing:

Reiki: This Japanese technique channels energy to promote relaxation, reduce stress, and facilitate healing. Practitioners believe it balances the body's energy centers.

Other Approaches:

Mind-Body Connection:

Counseling or Therapy: Mental and emotional health is integral to overall well-being. Therapy provides tools to cope with stress, manage emotions, and improve relationships.

Biofeedback: By gaining awareness and control over bodily functions, individuals can learn to manage conditions like chronic pain or anxiety.

Environmental Factors:

Detoxification: While controversial, some practices aim to support the body's natural detoxification processes. This might involve dietary changes, fasting, or specific treatments to eliminate toxins.

CHAPTER SEVEN

DIETARY ADJUSTMENTS FOR HEMORRHOID BLEEDING RELIEF

Hemorrhoids can be uncomfortable and distressing, especially when bleeding occurs. Making dietary adjustments can play a significant role in managing symptoms and providing relief. Here's a comprehensive guide to dietary adjustments for hemorrhoid bleeding:

Fiber Intake:

Increase Fiber: Aim for 25-30 grams of fiber per day. Fiber softens stools and eases bowel movements, reducing strain. Sources include fruits (apples, berries), vegetables (leafy greens, broccoli), whole grains (oats, brown rice), legumes (beans, lentils), and nuts/seeds (chia seeds, flaxseeds).

Supplements: If needed, consider fiber supplements like psyllium husk or methylcellulose, but ensure adequate water intake with these supplements.

Hydration:

Drink Plenty of Water: Staying hydrated softens stools, aiding smoother bowel movements. Aim for 8-10 cups of water per day.

Avoid Dehydrating Drinks: Minimize caffeine and alcohol intake as they can dehydrate the body, potentially worsening hemorrhoid symptoms.

Healthy Eating Habits:
Regular Meals: Stick to regular meal times to regulate bowel movements.

Smaller Portions: Overeating can lead to increased pressure on the rectum and aggravate hemorrhoids. Eat smaller, more frequent meals.

Foods to Include:

Fruits: Berries, apples, pears, prunes, and bananas.

Vegetables: Leafy greens, broccoli, Brussels sprouts, and carrots.

Whole Grains: Brown rice, whole-grain bread, quinoa, oats.

Legumes: Beans, lentils, chickpeas.

Healthy Fats: Avocado, nuts, seeds, and olive oil.

Foods to Limit or Avoid:

Spicy Foods: These can irritate the digestive system.

Processed Foods: High-fat, low-fiber processed foods can worsen constipation.

Dairy: Some individuals find dairy products exacerbate symptoms, so consider reducing intake to see if it helps.

Refined Grains: White bread, pastries, and processed cereals.

Fatty or Fried Foods: These can lead to harder stools and difficulty passing them.

Additional Tips:

Probiotics: Consider incorporating probiotic-rich foods (yogurt, kefir, sauerkraut) to promote gut health.

Gentle Exercise: Regular physical activity can aid digestion and alleviate constipation. Aim for at least 30 minutes of moderate exercise most days.

Don't Delay Bowel Movements: When you feel the urge, try not to postpone going to the bathroom.

Warm Baths: Soaking in a warm bath can help relax the anal muscles and alleviate discomfort.

Medical Advice:

Always consult with a healthcare professional for personalized advice. If bleeding persists or worsens despite dietary adjustments, seek medical attention promptly. In some cases, medical procedures or medications may be necessary for effective management.

CHAPTER EIGHT

EMBRACING WELLNESS: MIND-BODY PRACTICES TO ALLEVIATE HEMORRHOIDAL HEMORRHAGE

Hemorrhoids can be uncomfortable, so finding ways to manage them through mind-body practices can be beneficial. Mindfulness meditation can help reduce stress, which might alleviate some symptoms. Deep breathing exercises can also aid in relaxation and potentially reduce the discomfort associated with hemorrhoids. Yoga poses that focus on gentle stretching and promoting circulation might offer relief as well. Remember, though, it's essential to consult with a healthcare professional for proper medical advice and treatment.

Mindfulness Meditation:

Purpose: Mindfulness meditation aims to bring your attention to the present moment without judgment. Find a quiet and comfortable space to sit or lie down.

Close your eyes and focus on your breath. Notice the sensation of each inhale and exhale.

When your mind wanders (which is natural), gently bring your attention back to your breath.

Start with short sessions, gradually increasing the duration as you become more comfortable. Consistency is key; aim for daily practice.

Deep Breathing Exercises:

Purpose: Deep breathing helps activate the body's relaxation response, reducing stress and promoting a sense of calm.

- Find a comfortable seated or lying position.

- Inhale deeply through your nose, expanding your diaphragm.

- Exhale slowly and completely through your mouth or nose.

- Focus on making your breaths slow, deep, and rhythmic.

- Practice deep breathing for 5-10 minutes several times a day, especially during moments of stress.

Yoga:

Purpose: Yoga combines physical postures, breath control, and meditation to promote overall well-being.

- Choose gentle yoga poses that don't strain the affected area. Avoid intense inversions or positions that increase pressure on the rectal area.

- Incorporate poses like Child's Pose, Cat-Cow, and Legs Up the Wall, which can aid in relaxation and improve circulation.

- Pay attention to your body and modify poses as needed. If a pose causes discomfort, skip it.

- Include relaxation and meditation components at the end of your yoga session.

Additional Tips:

Hydration: Drink plenty of water to maintain soft and regular bowel movements, reducing strain during bowel movements.

Fiber-rich Diet: Consume a high-fiber diet with fruits, vegetables, and whole grains to prevent constipation.

Warm Baths: Soaking in a warm bath may help relax the muscles and alleviate discomfort.

Caution:

Always consult with a healthcare professional before starting a new wellness routine, especially if you have pre-existing health conditions.

If hemorrhoidal hemorrhage persists or worsens, seek medical attention promptly.

Combining these mind-body practices into your daily routine may contribute to managing the discomfort associated with hemorrhoids. However, it's crucial to approach these practices as complementary to medical advice and treatment, not as a substitute. Listen to your body, be consistent, and prioritize your well-being.

CONCLUSION

Hemorrhoids are common, but the discomfort and bleeding they cause can have a significant impact on your quality of life.

Unraveling Hemorrhoidal Hemorrhage: Exploring Hemorrhoidal Hemorrhage addresses this problem by recognizing the complex nature of hemorrhoids and considering both conventional medical approaches and complementary methods to effectively treat the condition.

We strive to provide a holistic perspective.

Diagnosis is the basis of effective hemorrhoid treatment.

It's important to understand the different types of internal and external hemorrhoids and their varying degrees of severity.

To diagnose and classify hemorrhoids, doctors use various methods such as visual examination, digital examination, and anoscopy.

These evaluations help determine the most appropriate treatment and management strategy.

However, prevention is an important pillar in the treatment of hemorrhoids.

Lifestyle changes play an important role in preventing the onset of the disease and reducing the likelihood of a disease flare-up.

Strategies such as maintaining a high-fiber diet, maintaining adequate fluid intake, avoiding prolonged sitting or straining during bowel movements, and regular exercise are important parts of preventive care.

Beyond traditional medical interventions, a holistic approach offers complementary options for treating hemorrhoid bleeding.

Herbal medicines such as witch hazel and aloe vera are known for their calming effects and are often used topically to relieve discomfort.

Sitz baths with warm water to soothe the affected area can also help relieve symptoms.

Additionally, dietary changes and supplementation with fiber, flavonoids, and bioflavonoids can help soften stool and reduce inflammation.

Taking probiotics also contributes to overall gut health, which can affect the severity of hemorrhoids.

Mind-body exercises such as yoga and meditation have potential benefits by reducing stress levels, which can indirectly affect hemorrhoid symptoms.

Stress management is increasingly recognized as an essential part of overall health, and its importance in treating conditions such as hemorrhoids should not be underestimated.

Additionally, alternative therapies such as acupuncture, which may relieve pain and improve blood circulation, are gaining attention and may be useful in treating hemorrhoid symptoms.

Although these holistic methods can provide relief, it is important to emphasize the importance of individualized care.

What works for one person may not be equally effective for another.

Therefore, an integrative approach that considers both traditional medical treatments and holistic treatments tailored to individual needs is often most beneficial.

Support groups and educational resources also play an important role in helping individuals cope with the emotional and psychological effects of hemorrhoids.

It is important to address the stigma with this condition and create an environment where individuals feel safe seeking advice and support.

As research progresses and our understanding of holistic therapies improves, the integration of these approaches into mainstream medical care may become more common.

Collaboration between traditional health care providers and physicians specializing in integrative medicine can further improve patient care and outcomes.

Ultimately, the study of hemorrhoid bleeding goes beyond physical symptoms to encompass the overall well-being of people affected by this disease.

By taking a comprehensive approach that combines medical expertise and holistic care, we are paving the way to more effective management strategies that address the complex nature of hemorrhoids and help people suffering from this common condition.

9 798886 954675